Contents

...a wheezing in Children

hanged

Simon Godfrey, MD, PhD, FRCP

Professor of Pediatrics
Director, Institute of Pulmonology
Hadassah University Hospital
Jerusalem, Israel

Peter J Barnes, MA, DM, DSc, FRCP

Professor of Thoracic Medicine
National Heart and Lung Institute
and Royal Brompton Hospital
London, UK

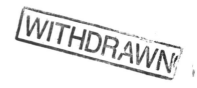
MARTIN DUNITZ

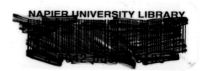

Although every effort has been made to ensure that the drug doses and other information are presented accurately in this publication, the ultimate responsibility rests with the prescribing physician. Neither the publishers nor the authors can be held responsible for errors or for any other consequences arising from the use of information contained herein.

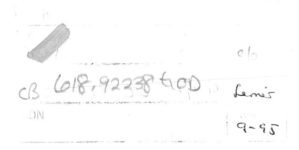

© Martin Dunitz Ltd 1997

First published in the United Kingdom
in 1997 by

Martin Dunitz Ltd
The Livery House
7– 9 Pratt Street
London NW1 0AE

A CIP record for this book is available
from the British Library.

ISBN 1-85317-394-0

Printed and bound in Spain by Cayfosa

Which diseases cause children to wheeze?

Wheezing and abnormally noisy breathing is one of the commonest respiratory symptoms in children and may be due to a wide variety of problems located in the respiratory pathways. Asthma is the commonest cause of generalized wheezing in children and bronchiolitis is the commonest cause in infants, but noisy breathing may also be due to a congenital anomaly, a genetic disorder, an acquired disease or a combination of these factors. The origin and characteristics of wheezing or noisy breathing depend to some degree on the underlying problem.

Site of the abnormal noise

- Nose, airways above the larynx
- Larynx, trachea and main bronchi
- Small bronchi and bronchioles
- Combination of these sites

Mechanism of abnormal noise

- Narrowing or distortion of the airway
- Bronchospasm
- Inflammation causing swelling of airway wall
- Secretions, aspiration
- Combination of processes

Timing and characteristics of noise

- Predominantly inspiratory
- Predominantly expiratory
- Stridulous and basically monophonic
- Musical and polyphonic

Many conditions affecting the small airways also result in excess secretion, coughing and the presence of crepitations (crackles) on examination. Some types of chronic obstructive pulmonary disease (COPD) in infants and children superficially resemble the chronic bronchitis and emphysema seen in adults. Because of all these possibilities the physician must always bear in mind that *"not all that wheezes is asthma"*.

The following is a brief description of the conditions associated with wheezing or noisy breathing in infants and children, according to the site of generation of the noise.

Upper airways

Adenoid hypertrophy Very common in infants and preschool children, causing snoring, postnasal drip and cough. If very severe and prolonged, this may cause serious airway obstruction with respiratory failure and cor pulmonale.

Congenital laryngeal stridor A relatively common group of congenital anomalies (including partial or complete vocal cord paralysis) producing inspiratory stridor and respiratory distress in the newborn and young infant.

Laryngotracheobronchitis (croup) Usually due to a viral infection in the infant or young child, producing inspiratory stridor that is typically worse at night. Some children have repeated attacks – this is known as spastic croup.

Vocal cord dysfunction Typically affects adolescents or young adults but can occur in younger children and is often misdiagnosed as asthma. The condition is due to an emotional disorder (probably hysterical) in which there is vocal cord adduction during inspiration and/or expiration.

Trachea and main bronchi

Congenital airway anomalies The commonest are tracheo-malacia or bronchomalacia in which the cartilage rings are not rigid and the airway is unduly floppy, resulting in retention of secretions, noisy breathing and a tendency to infection. Tracheo-oesophageal fistula is almost invariably associated with tracheomalacia.

Vascular rings (Figure 1) Some vascular rings are entirely innocuous, but complete rings surrounding the trachea such as those due to a double aortic arch or pulmonary artery sling are very likely to produce central noisy breathing and airway compression.

Aspiration Gastro-oesophageal reflux (GOR) is extremely common in otherwise perfectly healthy young infants but occasionally causes trouble. Some infants not only reflux but also aspirate gastric contents into the lungs, producing recurrent episodes of airway obstruction with generalized wheezing and sometimes with frank pneumonia.

Foreign-body aspiration Most common in the 1–3 year age group, especially in boys. It usually produces local bronchial obstruction with atelectasis, hyperinflation or pneumonia.

Haemangioma and other tumours Tumours causing airway obstruction and central airway noisy breathing are extremely rare in childhood. Bronchial adenoma is the commonest airway tumour in children (usually in adolescent girls), but it is more likely to cause haemoptysis or pneumonia than noisy breathing.

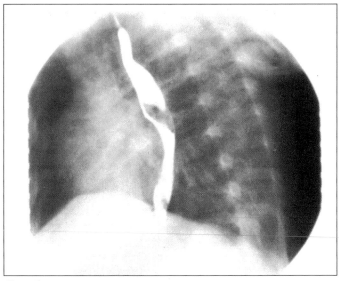

Figure 1
Lateral radiograph of barium swallow in a child with a vascular ring which caused compression of the trachea and oesophagus and is seen as an indent on the barium-filled oesophagus.

Small airways

Asthma Probably the most common significant chronic childhood disease in developed countries. The characteristic features of asthma in children include repeated attacks of airways obstruction with wheezing and/or coughing which subside spontaneously or in response to specific medication for asthma.

Acute viral bronchiolitis Very common in early infancy, occurring in winter epidemics mostly due to infection with the respiratory syncytial virus (RSV). The infant presents with respiratory distress, wheezing and hyperinflation which usually subsides spontaneously over a week or so.

Chronic post-bronchiolitic wheezing This affects up to 40% of infants following acute bronchiolitis. Infants have repeated episodes of wheezing which tend to become less severe and less frequent with time and cease after 2–3 years of age unless the child has classical asthma. The differentiation from asthma may be very difficult and, indeed, some believe that this is a form of true asthma.

Bronchiolitis obliterans An uncommon form of paediatric COPD with fixed airways obstruction and persistent wheezing which mostly follows severe viral pneumonia, often due to adenoviral infection. In some cases the disease may affect one lung far more than the other, resulting in a small hyperlucent lung. This is usually termed Swyer–James syndrome in the paediatric literature.

Bronchopulmonary dysplasia (BPD) A form of generalized COPD affecting mainly premature infants who have required intensive care with mechanical ventilation and high levels of inspired oxygen.

Primary ciliary dyskinesia The 'immotile cilia syndrome' affects a small proportion of children who suffer repeated respiratory infections, otitis media and sinusitis, but may present with a relatively mild form of COPD that is often mistaken for asthma or cystic fibrosis.

Cystic fibrosis (CF) An autosomal recessive disorder which in most patients causes severe and progressive lung disease and pancreatic insufficiency, and results in bronchiectasis. Infants with CF frequently present with a picture of COPD which is easily mistaken for bronchiolitis or asthma (Fig. 2).

Heart failure Heart failure often presents with variable or persistent wheezing due to small airways obstruction especially when there is a high pulmonary blood flow. A cardiac abnormality may not be obvious and the problem may be mistaken for asthma or postbronchiolitic wheezing.

Lung tissue

Congenital lobar emphysema One of the less rare developmental anomalies of lung tissue, in which one lobe or more is overinflated due to a pathological process leading to localized emphysema. The infant not infrequently presents with chronic wheezing.

Alpha-1 anti-trypsin deficiency This is a rare autosomal recessive inborn error of defence against damage by inflammatory changes, especially those induced by cigarette smoking, leading to a severe and generalized form of emphysema. The lung disease is extremely rare in infancy and childhood and normally only appears in early or middle adult life.

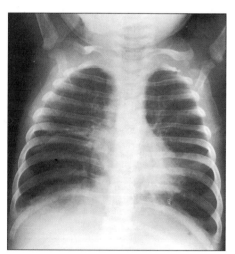

Figure 2
Chest radiograph of an infant with cystic fibrosis showing mild generalized hyperinflation and patchy infiltrates easily confused with asthma or simple bronchiolitis.

Pathophysiology of wheezing and noisy breathing

Mechanisms of wheezing and small airway noises

Wheezing and noise from the small airways are due to narrowing of the airway lumen and may be produced by several mechanisms:

- *Bronchoconstriction*: contraction of airway smooth muscle due to direct effects of inflammatory mediators (such as leukotrienes and histamine) or through activation of cholinergic nerves through reflex mechanisms
- *Airway wall thickening* due to oedema as a result of plasma exudation (acute), infiltration of inflammatory cells and deposition of extracellular matrix and increased bulk of airway smooth muscle (chronic). This results in excessive narrowing of the airways when airway smooth muscle contracts for geometric reasons (Fig. 3)
- *Increased secretions* (mucus, exuded plasma, inflammatory debris) in the airway lumen

Pathophysiology of asthma

The airways show a characteristic pathology which varies in intensity from mild to fatal asthma. Fibreoptic bronchial biopsies have shown that inflammation is present even in asymptomatic patients with mild asthma.

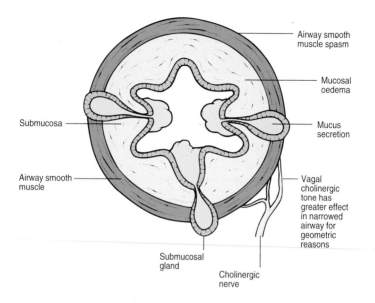

Figure 3
Airway narrowing in chronic obstructive pulmonary diseases.

- Infiltration with inflammatory cells (especially eosinophils and T-lymphocytes)
- Patchy epithelial shedding
- Airway smooth muscle thickening
- Subepithelial fibrosis (thickening of basement membrane)
- Mucus gland and goblet cell hyperplasia
- Widespread mucus plugging in severe/fatal asthma

Bronchial hyper-reactivity

Airway hyper-responsiveness caused by inflammation results in increased airway narrowing in response to a wide range of stimuli including mediators and physical stimuli. The characteristic pattern of inflammation involves activated mast cells, macrophages, eosinophils and T-helper lymphocytes ('chronic eosinophilic bronchitis'). Inflammatory cells release multiple inflammatory mediators (including histamine, leukotrienes, prostaglandins and bradykinin). Multiple intercellular messengers called cytokines are responsible for coordinating, amplifying and perpetuating the inflammatory response and attracting additional inflammatory cells.

Inflammatory mediators result in bronchoconstriction, mucus secretion, exudation of plasma and airway hyper-responsiveness (Fig. 4). Neural mechanisms may amplify the asthmatic inflammation (neurogenic inflammation).

Structural changes may occur with subepithelial fibrosis (basement membrane thickening), airway smooth muscle hyperplasia and new vessel formation (angiogenesis). These changes may underlie irreversible ('fixed') airflow obstruction.

Airway hyper-responsiveness results in airway narrowing due to bronchoconstriction in response to triggers, such as exercise, leading to wheezing and dyspnoea. Inflammation sensitizes sensory nerves in airways, resulting in cough and chest tightness.

Causes of asthma

Almost all children with asthma are *atopic* (having propensity to form IgE) and aeroallergens play an important role in driving the inflammatory disease. The underlying causes of asthma are not known. Atopy is inherited, but environmental mechanisms appear to be important in determining whether an atopic individual becomes an asthmatic. Several factors may increase the risks of developing asthma:

- Parental smoking and maternal smoking during pregnancy
- Exposure to a high concentration of allergens during infancy
- Viral infection during infancy

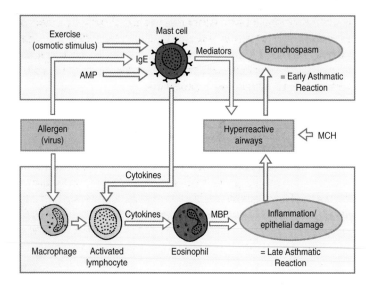

Figure 4

Diagrammatic representation of the mechanisms leading to early and late phase asthmatic reactions. The central abnormality is bronchial hyperreactivity which is the result of chronic asthmatic inflammatory changes and epithelial damage in the airways. When mast cells are stimulated allergically or by other means such as exercise or adenosine (AMP) they liberate mediators which cause bronchospasm (the early type of reaction). Allergic stimulation and other mechanisms (such as viral infection) can also initiate lymphocyte activation and cytokine release which leads to inflammatory infiltration (the late type of reaction) and epithelial damage in which eosinophils are involved. Hyperreactive airways from any cause, including for example COPD, can respond to direct stimulation by methacholine (MCH).

Bronchiolitis

Wheezing in viral bronchiolitis is probably due to inflammatory swelling in the wall of peripheral airways as a result of the inflammatory response to the virus infection. It is usually self-limiting, but may be of long duration with recurrent or persistent wheezing in the absence of new infection. Little is known about the inflammatory response, but recent studies of bronchoalveolar lavage suggest that this response involves macrophages, T-lymphocytes and neutrophils. There is evidence to suggest that infants with narrower airways may be more susceptible to developing bronchiolitis.

Bronchopulmonary dysplasia (BPD)

In BPD there is a fixed narrowing of the airways as a result of airway remodelling, scarring of the airways and deposition of collagen. The changes are due in part to respiratory distress syndrome in premature infants, in part to prolonged levels of high inspired oxygen and in part to barotrauma from positive pressure ventilation.

Cystic fibrosis (CF)

Wheezing in CF is predominantly due to increased mucus secretions in the airway lumen as a result of chronic infection (usually with *Pseudomonas spp*). There is an intense neutrophilic infiltration in the airway wall, with some inflammatory swelling, and this may underlie the increased airway responsiveness. Many of the inflammatory cytokines found in asthmatic inflammation can also be found in the airways of children with CF.

Primary ciliary dyskinesia (PCD)

In this condition there is a defect in the structure and movement of cilia of the lining epithelium throughout the respiratory tract as well as sperm immotility. In addition, there is retention of secretions and infection in the ear, paranasal sinuses and bronchi. In Kartaganer's syndrome, which is an extreme form of the PCD syndrome, there is also dextrocardia and bronchiectasis.

Other diseases with wheezing originating in small airways

The exact mechanism of wheezing in infants and children with gastro-oesophageal reflux and aspiration is uncertain – it may be due to local mechanical changes in the lungs or to reflex bronchospasm triggered by acid in the lower oesophagus. In heart failure, wheezing is presumably due to the compression of small airways by engorged blood vessels.

Mechanism of noisy breathing from large airways

Noisy breathing from the upper respiratory tract, trachea or large bronchi is due to the vibration of the walls adjacent to an obstruction during airflow. Changes in pressure during breathing may affect the diameter of even large airways so the noise may be prominent during inspiration (upper airways, larynx and extrathoracic trachea) or expiration (main bronchi) or both (some children with tracheomalacia). Because the obstruction is usually localized, the noise tends to be monophonic and localized centrally.

Differential diagnosis of wheezing in childhood

Recurrent or persistent wheezing or noisy breathing in infants or children may be due to many conditions (see pages 2–6) and therefore the differential diagnosis is important if the correct management is to be applied. Each condition has certain typical clinical features, changes on the plain chest radiograph and response to medication. This series of simple algorithms serves as a general guide to the correct diagnosis, but it should be borne in mind that there is considerable overlap and variation in how diseases affect children.

Most likely disorder – by age of onset of respiratory symptoms	
<1 year	
Premature infant	Bronchopulmonary dysplasia

Term newborn infant	Severe congenital airway anomalies
	    severe laryngomalacia
	    vocal cord paralysis
	    tracheal web
	Severe vascular rings
	    double aortic arch

Cont'd.

First 3 months of life	Congenital airway anomalies
	    laryngomalacia
	    tracheomalacia
	    bronchomalacia
	Vascular rings
	    aberrant subclavian artery
	Congenital lobar emphysema
	Viral bronchiolitis
	Aspiration
	Heart failure

First year of life	Postbronchiolitic wheeze True asthma – about 20% start <1 year Cystic fibrosis Aspiration Heart failure Viral bronchiolitis – less common Congenital anomalies – rare
> 1 year Pre-school child	Asthma Cystic fibrosis Primary ciliary dyskinesia Foreign body aspiration Croup Bronchiolitis obliterans Viral bronchiolitis – rare Aspiration – rare Congenital anomalies – very rare
Older child	Asthma Bronchiolitis obliterans Primary ciliary dyskinesia Foreign body aspiration – rare Cystic fibrosis – rare Endobronchial tumours – very rare

Most likely disorder – by natural history

Persistent from birth	Bronchopulmonary dysplasia (in the premature infant) Congenital anomalies of airway Vascular rings
Recent onset in healthy child	Viral bronchiolitis Croup Foreign-body aspiration
Persistent symptoms after acute illness	Bronchiolitis obliterans Foreign-body aspiration
Variable symptoms and symptom-free intervals	Asthma Postbronchiolitic wheezing Cystic fibrosis (unless severe) Primary ciliary dyskinesia Aspiration

Most likely disorder – by associated features

Premature birth	Bronchopulmonary dysplasia Asthma – possibly
Family history of asthma or allergy:	
yes	Asthma Spasmodic croup – sometimes
no	Bronchiolitis and all other conditions
Family history of chronic lung disease	Cystic fibrosis Primary ciliary dyskinesia
Onset in:	
winter	Bronchiolitis
autumn	Croup
Seasonal exacerbations	Asthma

Most likely disorder – by location and character of respiratory noise	
Central inspiratory stridor	Adenoid hypertrophy Congenital laryngeal stridor Croup Vocal cord paralysis
Central inspiratory and expiratory coarse noise	Tracheomalacia Vascular rings Foreign body (in trachea)
Coarse noise/wheeze over main bronchus	Bronchomalacia Foreign-body aspiration Aspiration – sometimes
Peripheral polyphonic musical wheezing usually over both lungs	Asthma Bronchiolitis Postbronchiolitic wheezing Cystic fibrosis (in infancy) Primary ciliary dyskinesia – sometimes Aspiration – sometimes Heart failure
Bilateral crepitations (crackles) ± wheezing	Asthma – especially in the infant Bronchiolitis Cystic fibrosis Primary ciliary dyskinesia Aspiration Heart failure

Most likely disorder – by simple chest radiograph	
X-ray essentially normal	Asthma – between attacks Bronchiolitis – between attacks Laryngeal disease Most congenital airway anomalies Most vascular rings Some foreign bodies
Generalized hyperinflation ± atelectasis/ infiltrates	Asthma Bronchiolitis COPD of all types

Localized hyperinflation	Foreign-body aspiration Isolated bronchomalacia Congenital lobar emphysema
Localized atelectasis or infiltrate	Asthma Aspiration Cystic fibrosis Foreign-body aspiration
Small unilateral hyperlucent lung	Bronchiolitis obliterans
Indentations in tracheal outline	Vascular rings

Most likely disorder – by response to medication

Selective β_2 bronchodilator response:	
good	Asthma – usually
mild	COPD of all types
none	All other diseases
Adrenaline response:	
good	Asthma – usually Croup – usually
mild	COPD – not usually tried
none	All other diseases
Corticosteroid response:	
good	Asthma
mild	COPD of all types
none	Croup Adenoid hypertrophy Acute bronchiolitis All other diseases
Diuretic response:	
good	Heart failure – if amenable to treatment
mild	Bronchopulmonary dysplasia
none	All other diseases

Expert help should be sought when there is:

- Uncertain diagnosis
- Failure to respond to treatment
- Failure to thrive
- Possible foreign-body aspiration
- Persistent or recurrent pneumonia
- Persistent chest radiographic changes
- Persistent or recurrent localized signs in the chest

Ancillary investigations

In most children with asthma, bronchiolitis and postbronchiolitic wheezing, the diagnosis can be made clinically with little or no ancillary investigations apart from a plain chest radiograph. However, it is very important not to miss an alternative diagnosis requiring different management just because wheezing is a common feature of asthma and bronchiolitis, and equally not to miss the diagnosis of asthma because the child presents with cough and fever which is attributed to pneumonia. Ancillary investigations are helpful in those patients whose diagnosis is uncertain.

There are a number of ancillary investigations available and the choice will obviously depend upon the patient's particular problem as well as on the child's ability to cooperate with the tests.

Tests of lung function

Spirometry and lung volumes

Indications:
- Diagnosis uncertain
- Management uncertain
- Evaluation of response to treatment
- Poor response to adequate treatment

There is a variety of sophisticated tests of lung function; the most informative and practical in children is a forced expiratory spirogram taken before and after the inhalation of a bronchodilator (Fig. 5).

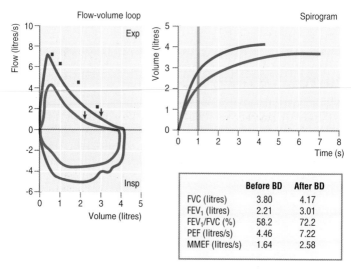

	Before BD	After BD
FVC (litres)	3.80	4.17
FEV_1 (litres)	2.21	3.01
FEV_1/FVC (%)	58.2	72.2
PEF (litres/s)	4.46	7.22
MMEF (litres/s)	1.64	2.58

Figure 5
Lung function in a patient with asthma. The blue lines are the baseline measurements, and the pink lines show improvement after inhalation of a bronchodilator (salbutamol 200 µg). Left panel shows flow-volume loops with inspiratory and expiratory records. Squares indicate the predicted normal value of the expiratory loop and arrows indicate the volume expired after one second. Right panel shows the expiratory spirogram for the same breath – the vertical mauve line indicates the volumes at one second. The results of the test are shown below and indicate generalized airflow obstruction with improvement (36% increase in FEV_1) after bronchodilator.

Forced vital capacity (FVC)

- Total volume that can be expelled during a maximal effort
- Should be normal except that in moderate to severe obstructive diseases gas trapping may prevent expiration to normal levels
- Very effort-dependent

Forced expired volume in 1 (FEV_1)

- Volume that is expelled in the first second of the forced expiration
- The most useful overall index of lung function
- Reflects the global severity of the airways obstruction
- Relatively independent of effort

Peak expiratory flow (PEF)

- Maximum expiratory flow achieved during forced expiration
- Very effort-dependent
- Quite reproducible in patients who cooperate fully
- Easy to measure at home
- Reflects chiefly the severity of obstruction in the larger airways
- Can be totally normal when the patient has marked small airways obstruction

Maximum mid-expiratory flow (MMEF)

- Maximum expiratory flow when half of the forced vital capacity has been expelled
- Sometimes called the forced expiratory flow at 50% of expiration, FEF_{50}
- Largely independent of effort
- Reflects chiefly the severity of the obstruction in the smaller airways
- May well be abnormal when the PEF and even the FEV_1 are normal

Forced expiratory flow at resting lung volume in infants (VmaxFRC)

- Simplest and most practical test of lung function in infants
- Jacket surrounding chest is suddenly inflated for 1–2 seconds
- Forced expiratory flow reduced in obstructive lung diseases
- Similar to the MMEF in older children

Plethysmography

- Measures airway resistance and lung volumes
- Rarely needed (or even practical) in young children
- Can be useful in older children when there is doubt about the diagnosis
- Plethysmography for infants aged 0–18 months is possible in specialized centres

Tests of bronchial reactivity by inhalation

Indications:
- Diagnosis uncertain
- Management uncertain

Age suitability:
- 6–8 years and older by lung function
- 3–6 years by breath sound/pulse oximetry
- 0–18 months by infant lung function tests

Bronchial challenge tests are used to detect the presence of bronchial hyper-reactivity. They are most useful when diagnosis of asthma is in doubt.

- Absence of bronchial hyper-reactivity virtually excludes the diagnosis of asthma
- Bronchial hyper-reactivity to methacholine or histamine is common to a number of chronic lung diseases besides asthma, including cystic fibrosis, bronchiolitis obliterans, primary ciliary dyskinesia and sometimes chronic infection
- May persist in children who have grown out of their asthma
- Recent studies have shown that bronchial hyper-reactivity to adenosine 5'-monophosphate is highly specific for asthma in children, but this test is not yet generally available

Histamine, methacholine or adenosine challenge is performed by having the child inhale increasing concentrations of the agent, usually during tidal breathing, and determining the concentration which causes a 20% fall in FEV_1 (PC_{20}). Values of <8 mg/ml for methacholine or histamine suggest airway hyper-reactivity.

Bronchial challenge tests can be performed in small children from about 3 years of age by the 'breath sound method' in which the child inhales increasing concentrations of the agent during tidal breathing. The physician determines the end-point by hearing the appearance of wheezing or crepitations on auscultation, by the appearance of persistent coughing or by the appearance of definite tachycardia or modest desaturation determined by pulse oximetry. An alternative to auscultation is the use of transcutaneous oxygen tension measurement to determine the end-point, but this requires expensive, delicate equipment.

In infants under 12–18 months of age, bronchial challenge tests can be performed using the thoracic compression technique to determine the end-point (normally a 40% fall in $V_{max}FRC$), but this is only available in highly specialized centres.

Testing for bronchial reactivity by exercise

Indications:
- Diagnosis uncertain
- Management uncertain

Age suitability:
- 6–7 years and older

Exercise challenge is also a highly specific method of demonstrating bronchial hyper-reactivity in asthmatics in whom 6–8 minutes of relatively hard running or cycling cause a fall of more than 10% in FEV_1. The child should breathe relatively dry air at room temperature since warm humid air reduces the response. About 70% of asthmatic children will develop exercise-induced asthma (EIA) which usually reaches its peak about 5 minutes after the end of exercise. This type of challenge is very useful in the older child or adolescent in whom EIA may be the only manifestation of asthma.

Imaging

Indications:
- Diagnosis uncertain

Age suitability:
- All ages

Infants and children with wheezing or noisy breathing in whom the diagnosis is not obvious will often need some type of imaging, if the plain chest radiograph is unhelpful, or to clarify an abnormality seen on the plain film.

- Barium swallow is used to demonstrate oesophageal (and, by implication, tracheal) compression by an aberrant vessel or vascular ring; suspected gastro-oesophageal reflux with aspiration
- Computerized tomography of the chest will be needed if a vascular anomaly is suspected, and should be performed with the injection of contrast material
- Lung scintigraphy after the inhalation or injection of radioactive material can be helpful in demonstrating the site and severity of localized gas trapping such as occurs in congenital lobar emphysema
- Isotopic scanning after the ingestion of labelled milk is used to demonstrate gastro-oesophageal reflux and aspiration, but the results are generally very unreliable

Bronchoscopy

Indications:
- Diagnosis uncertain

Age suitability:
- All ages

Flexible fibreoptic bronchoscopy can readily be safely performed with light sedation and topical anaesthesia on an outpatient basis in almost all infants and children. In experienced hands paediatric fibreoptic bronchoscopy yields clinically meaningful information in some 90% of investigations. The indications for bronchoscopy in a child with wheezing or abnormally noisy breathing are:

- Possible foreign-body aspiration (definite foreign-body aspiration requires rigid bronchoscopy under general anaesthesia)
- To determine the site of the lesion in congenital or acquired abnormalities of the nasopharynx, larynx and large airways (Fig. 6)
- To perform bronchoalveolar lavage if infection or aspiration is suspected

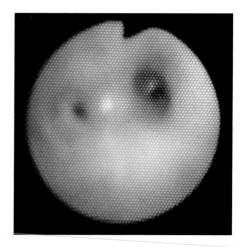

Figure 6
Photograph through fibreoptic bronchoscope showing stenosis of left main bronchus in an infant with noisy breathing initially referred with a diagnosis of asthma.

A timely bronchoscopy of this type may well save the child from large amounts of unnecessary irradiation, other unnecessary investigations and unnecessary treatment with medications for asthma or antibiotics.

Oesophageal pH measurement

Indications:
- Diagnosis uncertain

Age suitability:
- All ages

Wheezing due to gastro-oesophageal reflux can be very difficult to diagnose and is resistant to treatment with medication for asthma. The demonstration of an abnormal amount of reflux for the age of the child by overnight measurement of pH with a probe in the oesophagus can help make the diagnosis.

Allergy testing

Indications:
- Diagnosis uncertain
- Management uncertain
- Allergy testing is necessary to characterize the child as atopic

Age suitability:
- Mainly older children

Almost all children with asthma are atopic and so the inability to demonstrate IgE-mediated allergy may cast doubt on the diagnosis.

- *Skin prick testing* is used to document atopy and identify possible allergens. The most likely allergens are domestic mites, cockroaches, cat and dog fur, grass pollen, *Aspergillus fumigatus*. In infants, cows' milk and eggs might be important, mainly in children with concomitant atopic dermatitis
- *RAST* determines specific IgE in blood and is indicated only when skin testing is not possible (e.g. in severe eczema) and when the child is more frightened of the skin test than of a blood test
- *Blood eosinophilia or elevated total IgE* is often absent in children with asthma and may be present in children with intestinal parasites, so that these tests are rarely helpful
- *Allergen inhalation bronchial challenge* is not used routinely in children because of the danger of severe reactions and side-effects

Ambulatory monitoring of asthma

Indications:
- Management uncertain
- Evaluation of response to treatment
- Poor response to adequate treatment

Age suitability:
- Diaries – all ages
- PEF meter – older children (>6 years)

Almost all children with asthma can and should be managed on an ambulatory basis in their own home. In order to help evaluate the severity of the disease and its response to treatment on a day-to-day basis, the parents or an older child can be provided with an asthma diary (see pages 76–77).

Recently, great emphasis has been placed on the continuous or periodic use of PEF meters at home by all adults with chronic asthma, with treatment guidelines being based on the value recorded and the diurnal variation. Older children can use these devices as well as (or better than) adults. However, all but the most obsessive patients find this irksome and most soon abandon regular recording.

Other investigations to aid in diagnosis

A sweat test can be easily performed in any child except newborn infants. Elevated sweat sodium/chloride is diagnostic of cystic fibrosis, although this may be normal or borderline in rare genetic variants.

CF transmembrane receptor (CFTR) genetic studies have shown that the cystic fibrosis genotype can be identified in a blood sample. Almost all genetic variants of CFTR can be identified in specialized centres.

Respiratory tract cilia have an abnormal structure on electron microscopy in primary ciliary dyskinesia (PCD) syndrome. A biopsy may be taken from the nasal mucosa as representative of cilia throughout the bronchial tree. Cilia move abnormally in PCD, as seen qualitatively under light microscopy on fresh specimen. Quantitative measurement is also possible, but complicated.

Managing asthma

Many conditions can cause children to wheeze or breathe noisily; the most common of these is bronchial asthma. Children with asthma usually respond very well to treatment and almost all should be able to lead full normal lives, apart from the need for appropriate medication. The greatest problems with asthma in young children are:

- Failure to diagnose asthma in a child whose main symptom is cough, especially at night or after exertion
- Misdiagnosis of asthma as recurrent pneumonia because attacks are frequently precipitated by febrile (viral) illnesses. Note: true recurrent pneumonia in a child is rare and almost always indicates a serious underlying condition (e.g. CF, foreign body, immune deficiency etc.). Asthma should always be considered in a child with recurrent lower respiratory tract disease, especially when there are definite symptom-free intervals between attacks
- Evaluation of disease activity usually depends on the impression of a third party who does not see the child for most of the day
- Unreliable/reluctant use of PEF meters by young/older children
- Need to give medications by inhalation which may present practical difficulties with inhalation devices and problems with timing of medication in children at school
- Anxiety of parents (and some doctors) about unwanted side-effects of treatment leading to suboptimal treatment and limitation of everyday activities
- True adverse effects of the disease or its treatment on normal growth and development

Internationally accepted guidelines for the management of asthma in children have been modified by paediatricians to take account of the special problems of treating asthma in children.

Clinical evaluation of severity of asthma

In most cases, the assessment of the clinical severity of asthma should be based on the following criteria, which reflect the amount of disturbance to the everyday life of the child or family. It is only practical to consider the 12 months before evaluation.

- Number of daytime attacks lasting more than 24 hours and needing extra medication
- Presence of completely symptom-free intervals lasting more than 4 weeks without medication
- Frequency of waking at night because of asthma symptoms
- Amount of absence from school or other child care facility because of asthma
- Ability of the child to keep up with peers in normal physical activity
- Number and type of medications required on a regular daily basis
- Frequency of use of extra relief medications on an as-needed basis
- Frequency of hospital admissions or Accident and Emergency Department attendances
- Frequency of any life-threatening episodes of acute asthma requiring intensive care

On the basis of this information, the severity of asthma can be divided into three broad groups, although any categorization will depend upon the symptom tolerance of the patient:

Mild intermittent asthma

- Attacks requiring infrequent medication with long symptom-free periods
- Ratio of symptom-free to symptomatic days of at least 10 : 1
- Child should not lose more than the occasional day from school
- Sleep should be undisturbed most nights
- Normal physical activity can be taken
- Extra medication may be needed if exercise-induced asthma is a problem
- Asthma can usually be managed with medication on an as-needed basis

Moderate persistent asthma

- Child unwell more often than well
- Some absence from school is usual
- Nocturnal symptoms are common
- Exercise is often problematic
- May be less symptomatic if child is receiving appropriate medication
- Asthma can usually be controlled with modest doses of medication on a regular basis

Severe persistent asthma

- Daily or very frequent symptoms
- Sleep is disturbed most nights
- Child cannot exercise normally
- Child is prone to miss school
- May be less symptomatic if child is receiving appropriate medication
- Requires continuous medication in relatively large doses to control symptoms
- Need to attend physician or hospital clinic at frequent intervals

A distinction must be drawn between the overall clinical severity of asthma, as defined above, and the severity of individual exacerbations during the course of the disease. Children with mild or moderate asthma may occasionally have a severe attack but this does not mean that they are severe asthmatics, as defined by the amount of disturbance to their everyday life. Even in moderate or severe asthma there are often seasonal exacerbations and remissions which may require changes in regular medication.

In addition to the three groups described above, there are two special subgroups of asthma relevant to children:

Exercise-induced asthma (EIA)

- Exercise is a potent stimulus for a short attack of bronchospasm (Fig.7)
- EIA occurs in almost all asthmatics if they exercise hard enough
- Some children, mostly fit young adolescents, have little or no clinical asthma on a day-to-day basis but may be severely handicapped by EIA when they take part in sports – these children can easily be dismissed as neurotic if the appropriate tests are not performed

Figure 7
Typical exercise-induced asthma (EIA) in a child. During the 6 minutes of exercise there is a small improvement in lung function. Lung function begins to fall at the end of exercise and the attack of EIA reaches its greatest severity 5 minutes after the end of exercise.

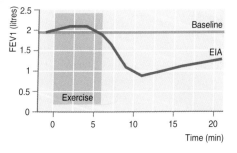

Sudden life-threatening asthma

- A few asthmatics suffer from infrequent but devastatingly severe attacks of asthma
- Attacks often require admission to an intensive care unit and ventilatory support
- It is not uncommon for the patient to be totally symptom-free in the intervals between attacks
- These children present a very high-risk group and their management is problematical

Choice of therapy

This depends on:

- Amount of disturbance to the everyday life of the child and/or their family
- Response of the disease to the treatment prescribed
- Ability of the child and/or family to comply with the prescribed treatment
- Avoidance of undesirable side-effects of treatment

The continuing management of the patient requires a periodic review to determine whether the treatment plan prescribed in accordance with these principles achieves the goals of good control of asthma. Treatment may need to be changed and this is best done in a controlled, stepwise fashion.

Change of treatment during follow up

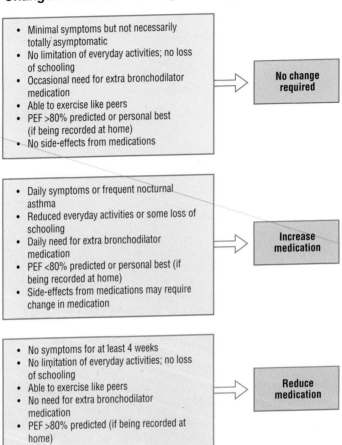

- Minimal symptoms but not necessarily totally asymptomatic
- No limitation of everyday activities; no loss of schooling
- Occasional need for extra bronchodilator medication
- Able to exercise like peers
- PEF >80% predicted or personal best (if being recorded at home)
- No side-effects from medications

No change required

- Daily symptoms or frequent nocturnal asthma
- Reduced everyday activities or some loss of schooling
- Daily need for extra bronchodilator medication
- PEF <80% predicted or personal best (if being recorded at home)
- Side-effects from medications may require change in medication

Increase medication

- No symptoms for at least 4 weeks
- No limitation of everyday activities; no loss of schooling
- Able to exercise like peers
- No need for extra bronchodilator medication
- PEF >80% predicted (if being recorded at home)

Reduce medication

Which medication for which child?

The generally accepted guidelines to asthma management in children are based on a stepwise approach to management (Fig. 8). Initially it may be necessary to give a short course of relatively intensive treatment to 'de-wheeze' the child and then continue at the step most appropriate to the initial severity of asthma (see above) and progress to the next step when control cannot be achieved, providing medication is being used correctly. Once control has been maintained for several months, treatment should be stepped down so that the patient is maintained on the minimum treatment needed for optimal control.

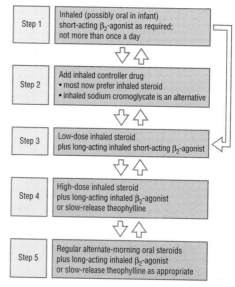

Figure 8
Step-wise approach to asthma therapy. Patients should increase the treatment until control is achieved. Patients may start at any step depending on the level of severity. Once control is achieved patients should step-down treatment.

Step 1 — Inhaled (possibly oral in infant) short-acting β_2-agonist as required; not more than once a day

Step 2 — Add inhaled controller drug
• most now prefer inhaled steroid
• inhaled sodium cromoglycate is an alternative

Step 3 — Low-dose inhaled steroid plus long-acting inhaled short-acting β_2-agonist

Step 4 — High-dose inhaled steroid plus long-acting inhaled β_2-agonist or slow-release theophylline

Step 5 — Regular alternate-morning oral steroids plus long-acting inhaled β_2-agonist or slow-release theophylline as appropriate

A major factor in the management of asthma in children is the ability of the child to take medications, especially inhaled medications, and the ability of the parents to administer them to their child. It is quite useless to prescribe a metered dose inhaler without a spacer for most young children and quite unrealistic to expect parents to administer medications through a nebulizer to a screaming infant who is terrified by the noise of the compressor. Details of the devices available and alternative medications suitable for children of different ages and different temperaments are given on pages 67–74 and the recommended doses are listed in the Appendix.

Step 1: inhaled β_2 -agonist as required

- Use a short-acting β_2-agonist (e.g. salbutamol, terbutaline) as required for symptom relief – usually 1–2 puffs
- Oral preparations may be tried in mild cases but the inhaled route is preferable for all children
- If treatment is required more than once daily, move to step 2 after ensuring the child has a good inhaler technique
- Concerns have been expressed about regular use of short-acting inhaled β_2-agonists

Step 2: regular inhaled anti-inflammatory drugs

- Add a regular anti-inflammatory agent as preventative (prophylactic) medication
- Paediatricians usually consider that inhaled sodium cromoglycate 3–4 times daily to be the treatment of choice in children as this drug is entirely without side-effects. Many parents find this regimen very inconvenient
- Increasing confidence in the use of inhaled corticosteroids in children means that many physicians now prefer to use these drugs as first-line preventative therapy. Start with a higher dose (400–600 µg bd for beclomethasone or budesonide, 200–300 µg for fluticasone) and reduce it once control is achieved
- There is little or no justification for continuing sodium cromoglycate if the child is receiving an inhaled corticosteroid
- A 5-day course of oral corticosteroid such as prednisone or betamethasone (which tastes better) should be given at the start of treatment if the child is significantly obstructed

Step 3: low-dose inhaled steroids plus long-acting inhaled β_2 -agonist

- Continue with an inhaled corticosteroid
- Add a long-acting β_2-agonist such as salmeterol or formoterol
- An inhaled short acting β_2-agonist should be used in addition on an as-needed basis up to a maximum of 3–4 times per 24 hours

Step 4: high-dose inhaled steroids and bronchodilators

- Increase inhaled steroids up to 1000 µg daily of beclomethasone or budesonide (and half this amount of fluticasone) for younger children and 1500 µg for older children
- The use of an appropriate valved spacer or a dry powder inhalation device is recommended. Advise mouth-washing when a dry powder inhaler is used
- Continue with a long-acting inhaled β_2-agonist such as salmeterol or formoterol
- Alternative is to add regular slow-release oral theophylline on a twice daily basis – not popular (except in the United States) because of side-effects
- Some evidence suggests theophylline may have anti-inflammatory properties in lower doses than traditionally prescribed
- Inhaled short acting β_2-agonist should be used in addition on an as-needed basis up to a maximum of 3–4 times per 24 hours
- Ipratropium or oxitropium bromide can be combined with the β_2-agonist if desired

Step 5: regular alternate morning oral corticosteroids

- If child cannot be controlled on inhaled corticosteroids even in high dose, first consider whether
  - (a) the inhalation technique is inadequate
  - (b) the medication is not being taken for some reason
- Oral corticosteroid prophylaxis is indicated
  - (c) if it is impossible to control the asthma with an adequate dose of corticosteroid inhaled by a correct technique
  - (d) if it is clear that this goal is unattainable (some children/parents hate all inhalers)
- Give about 1.0 mg/kg of prednisolone or 0.1 mg/kg of betamethasone (which most children seem to prefer) every other morning
- There is little or no point in persisting with the inhaled corticosteroid under such circumstances
- Additional medications should be used as in step 4 as appropriate

Cont'd.

- In exceptionally severe, steroid-resistant asthma, consider methotrexate, oral gold or cyclosporin A as a way to reduce the dose of oral steroid. However, there is very little experience with these potentially hazardous therapies in children

Step-down

Once control is achieved, treatment should be reviewed every 1–2 months initially and at longer intervals as experienced is gained with the individual child. Stepwise reduction of treatment may be possible if the patient:

- Has been virtually symptom-free
- Requires little or no rescue additional bronchodilator medication for 1–2 months

Children with markedly seasonal variations in asthma severity may need to vary their treatment according to the season.

When to refer to a specialist clinic

A child should be referred to a specialist clinic if there is doubt about diagnosis (see pages 13–18) or if their asthma is difficult to control. This group of patients includes:

- Children requiring high-dose inhaled steroids
- Children with brittle asthma
- Children or their parents with compliance or psychological problems
- Children who have recently been discharged from hospital
- Children who require maintenance oral steroids

Management of exercise-induced asthma (EIA)

EIA is most common in fit young adolescents and adults who take part in vigorous sports. The problem can be avoided or dealt with by recommending appropriate types of exercise and appropriate medication. Asthmatics should be encouraged to take part in normal physical activities; a significant number of Olympic gold medallists have active asthma and certain medications (short acting β_2-agonists, inhaled corticosteroids, cromones) are allowed by international sports regulatory boards. Under no circumstances should children be kept off usual games for fear of EIA – they should receive appropriate treatment. However, the risks of EIA under adverse circumstances such as during scuba diving should be seriously considered when choosing a sporting activity.

Conditions most likely to cause an attack of EIA are:

- 6–8 minutes of continuous hard exercise breathing cold or dry air
- Exercise during the allergy season in allergic asthmatics
- Failure to take appropriate medication

Conditions least likely to cause an attack of EIA include:

- Intermittent exercise, e.g. many team games
- Swimming or other exercise breathing warm humid air
- Appropriate premedication used

Medication for EIA

- Most effective treatment is premedication with a short-acting inhaled β_2-agonist bronchodilator 5 minutes before exercise
- Inhaled corticosteroids and cromones (sodium cromoglycate, nedocromil sodium) may somewhat blunt the severity of EIA
- Corticosteroid or cromone prophylaxis is not indicated if the sole manifestation of asthma is EIA
- Inhaled β_2-agonist bronchodilators, inhaled corticosteroids and cromones are sanctioned for use by asthmatic athletes

Management of an acute attack of asthma

Every year, children with asthma die of their disease and from analyses of the circumstances it appears that the large majority (over 80%) of such deaths are avoidable. They result either from incompetent management of acute exacerbations, or from negligence on the part of the family. The correct management of acute exacerbations of asthma (Fig. 9) is essential if this mortality is to be avoided and depends upon the following:

For ambulatory patients

- Correct interpretation of warning symptoms at home
- Correct treatment at home
- Recognition when hospital treatment is needed

For children coming to hospital

- Correct evaluation in Accident and Emergency Department
- Correct treatment in Accident and Emergency Department
- Recognition when transfer to intensive care is needed
- Correct timing of discharge from hospital

For all patients

- Correct follow-up and modification of treatment

Non-life-threatening asthma

Symptoms and signs
- Child is too breathless to talk normally
- Tachypnoea >50 breaths/minute
- Tachycardia >140 beats/minute
- PEF (rarely available in children) <50% predicted

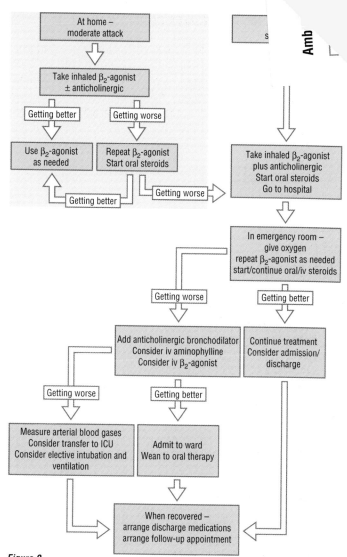

Figure 9

Algorithm for the management of acute asthma, the details of which are amplified in the text. The management shown surrounded by the tinted area in the upper left corner relates to moderate acute asthma not requiring hospitalization unless it is unresponsive to treatment at home.

Step 1
- Nebulized β_2-agonist ± anticholinergic if nebulizer is available
- MDI + spacer β_2-agonist ± anticholinergic is good alternative

Step 2
- Feeling better – repeat bronchodilator every 2–4 hours until back to usual state
- No better – repeat step 1 after 20 minutes and if still no better, move to

Step 3
- Start oral steroids (beginning of 3–5 day course) and repeat bronchodilator after 20 minutes
- If no better, consider going straight to hospital or calling an ambulance

Potentially life-threatening attack

Symptoms and signs
- Cyanosis of lips or tongue
- Confusion, coma or agitation
- Exhaustion, feeble respiratory effort
- PEF (if available) <33% predicted or best

The patient should be given the recommended treatment and taken straight to hospital.

Treatment at home and on way to hospital

- Oxygen if available
- Nebulized β_2-agonist combined with anticholinergic (ipratropium bromide), if nebulizer available, or
- MDI + spacer β_2-agonist and anticholinergic (ipratropium bromide)
- First dose of oral prednisolone

Evaluation in Accident and Emergency Department

- History of present illness and all medications taken in past 24 hours
- Quick relevant physical examination (cyanosis, retractions, air entry)
- Peak flow measurement if possible (unlikely in young children)
- Tachycardia and tachypnea suggests severe asthma
- Bradycardia, hypotension suggest severe asthma
- Pulse oximetry – saturation <90% on room air suggests severe asthma
- Urgent chest radiograph if pneumothorax suspected but *do not delay treatment*
- Arterial blood gas analysis if asthma thought to be severe

Treatment in Accident and Emergency Department

Step 1
- Oxygen by face mask to keep saturation >95%
- Nebulized β_2-agonist combined with anticholinergic (ipratropium bromide)
- As alternative, use MDI + spacer β_2-agonist and ipratropium bromide plus
- Oral prednisolone if child relatively well and willing and able to swallow medications

  or
- Methylprednisolone/ hydrocortisone intravenously

If the patient improves, progress to

Step 2a
- Oxygen as needed
- Repeat bronchodilator every 2–4 hours
- Oral/i.v. corticosteroids once daily (6-hourly dosing is traditional but unnecessary)
- Monitor heart rate, respiratory rate and saturation

Continuing improvement, progress to

Step 2b

- Stop intravenous therapy
- Regular inhaled bronchodilators
- Oral corticosteroids once daily (twice daily dosing is traditional but unnecessary)
- Consider discharge and changes in regular medication

If the patient does not improve after step 1, progress to

Step 3

- Add nebulized anticholinergic if not already being used
- Nebulized bronchodilators every 20 minutes
- Consider i.v. aminophylline (only maintenance dose if patient takes theophylline preparations at home)
- Consider i.v. β_2-agonist
- Repeat blood gas measurement
- Measure theophylline level if aminophylline is being used
- Measure electrolytes and glucose
- Beware of inappropriate ADH secretion – do not overload with fluids

Consider moving the patient to intensive care if:

- Becoming tired with weak respiratory effort
- Becoming comatosed
- Arterial PO_2 <60 mmHg (<8 kPa) or saturation <90% on >60% inspired O_2
- Arterial PCO_2 >45 mmHg (> 6 kPa)

Remember that elective intubation and ventilation is always better than an emergency procedure. *Never give sedatives* unless the patient is intubated and ventilated. When the child starts improving with or without a period of ventilation, continue with steps 2a and 2b.

Discharge and follow-up

Criteria for discharge from hospital
- Symptom-free or return to usual ambulatory condition
- Good air entry and wheeze-free on examination
- PEF >75% predicted or personal best if it can be measured
- Saturation >92% breathing room air
- Full understanding by child and/or family of medications to be taken
- Ability to use any prescribed inhaler device correctly
- Discharge medications being taken correctly while still in hospital
- Adequately supportive home conditions

Discharge medications should include:

- Steadily reducing course of oral corticosteroids over about 1 week
- Regular inhaled bronchodilators until completely symptom-free, then as needed
- Increased dose of inhaled corticosteroids for 2–3 weeks if taken before admission
- Consider starting prophylaxis if not used before admission

Discharge arrangements should include:

- Adequate discharge summary for family physician
- Follow-up appointment for respiratory outpatient clinic within 1–2 weeks
- Written self-management 'action plan' (revised if necessary)
- Asthma symptom diary if considered necessary
- PEF meter to use regularly at home if considered necessary (unusual)
- Attempt to avoid contact with any overt asthma-precipitating factors

Acute viral bronchiolitis

No medications have consistently been shown to alter the course of acute RSV bronchiolitis. Treatment is supportive, with added oxygen if necessary. Some recent studies have shown improvement in symptoms after the inhalation of adrenaline which, unlike the selective 2 bronchodilators, is also a vasoconstrictor and may reduce congestion of the bronchial walls. Many studies have shown that corticosteroids are not effective in acute RSV bronchiolitis, even when given systemically. In severe cases the infant may progress to respiratory failure and require mechanical ventilation.

The antiviral agent ribavirin will combat RSV infections but has only been tried by the inhaled route in infants at very high risk such as premature infants or those with severe congenital heart disease. Administration of ribavirin by inhalation is very cumbersome and not without some theoretical risk to the medical and nursing staff attending the patient. Hyperimmune RSV gammaglobulin has also been shown to be effective in preventing RSV infection in very-high-risk infants but has not yet been shown to help in the infant who has already been infected.

While no hard rules can be given as to management, the following scheme gives some indication as to the severity of the problem and likely management.

Mild
- Infant taking feeds well
- Mild tachypnea (<40/min)
- Mild respiratory distress (mild intercostal retractions)
- Not clinically hypoxic
- Treat at home – review if child deteriorates

Moderate
- Poor feeding
- Moderate tachypnea (>40/min)
- Moderate respiratory distress (widespread retractions)
- Moderate hypoxia in air (saturation >85%)
- Admit to hospital, oxygen by hood, intravenous fluids

Severe
- Refusal to feed
- Marked respiratory distress (tachypnea >60 and/or severe retractions)
- Marked hypoxia in air (saturation <85%)
- Respiratory failure ($PaCO_2$ > 40 mmHg)
- Admit to intensive care unit, consider intubation and mechanical ventilation
- Consider ribavirin gamma globulin

Recurrent post-bronchiolitic wheezing

Following an initial attack of presumed RSV bronchiolitis during the winter epidemic, a considerable number of infants continue to wheeze intermittently in a fashion which closely resembles asthma in older children and indeed may well be a virus-induced form of asthma. This differs from the usual type of childhood asthma in its onset in early infancy and its tendency to become less severe and cease at a relatively young age.

The management of this condition is problematic. It is almost irresistible to try anti-asthma medication for the recurrent post-bronchiolitic wheezy infant, and occasionally they seem to respond. A trial of therapy should be attempted if symptoms are severe enough to distress the infant or the family. The child should be given an inhaled corticosteroid on a twice-daily basis with an additional inhaled bronchodilator on an as-needed basis up to 3–4 times daily.

If no response is obtained in 1–2 weeks, it is probably not worth persisting with the corticosteroid. Other agents such a sodium cromoglycate are unlikely to help in this type of infant.

It is always important to remember that chronic respiratory symptoms in infancy may be due to other serious diseases including cystic fibrosis. *Beware of the chesty infant with failure to thrive.*

Management of the postbronchiolitic wheezy infant must include providing the parents with an explanation of the problem in terms they can understand:

- Explain the aetiology and epidemiology of bronchiolitis to the parents
- Reassure them that most infants recover and do not continue as asthmatics
- Explain that there is no cure other than time and that most infants recover completely

---

Viral croup

- In most children, no treatment is needed and the condition resolves within 2–3 days
- Inhalations of adrenaline help in those who are more seriously affected
- Oral or nebulized inhaled corticosteroids have been shown to lessen symptoms and shorten the course of the disease

---

- Very occasionally endotracheal intubation and intensive care will be needed
- Beware the child who appears to be desperately ill – croup due to acute bacterial epiglottitis may be extremely dangerous

Chronic obstructive pulmonary disorders

Cystic fibrosis

Management of CF is based on the prevention and treatment of respiratory infections with appropriate antibiotic therapy and physiotherapy:

- Pancreatic insufficiency is controlled with appropriate enzyme replacement therapy and vitamin supplementation
- Bronchodilators may be helpful in CF patients who have marked bronchial lability related to infection and chronic inflammatory changes in the airways
- Some infants with CF present with COPD closely resembling bronchiolitis and may even require mechanical ventilation
- Corticosteroids have been tried both for prophylaxis and for acute therapy in CF but the results are not clear-cut
- A trial of oral corticosteroid therapy should be undertaken in those with marked small airways obstruction

Primary ciliary dyskinesia

Children with PCD generally suffer from milder respiratory infections from an older age than children with CF. They do not have pancreatic insufficiency, but do have serious recurrent otitis media and sinusitis. Treatment is basically with antibiotics for any respiratory, ear or sinus infections, and bronchodilators may be used as an adjunct to respiratory physiotherapy (there is no evidence that corticosteroids help these patients). The prognosis is generally good.

Bronchiolitis obliterans

Bronchiolitis obliterans is a type of COPD due to severe damage to the small airways following a viral infection, usually with the adenovirus. The disease may virtually be confined to one lung which is left small and hyperlucent. It can also occur after lung transplantation, and is a major cause of death in transplanted patients. The clinical picture resembles severe bronchial asthma except that there are only minor fluctuations in the severity of the disease. There is little or no evidence of response to either bronchodilators or corticosteroids. Treatment is therefore supportive and it is important that the child should not suffer from the side-effects of unnecessary and unhelpful corticosteroid therapy. There is a tendency for the disease to improve with time.

Bronchopulmonary dysplasia

This type of COPD follows mechanical ventilation in premature infants. It may vary greatly in severity from infant to infant, with a natural tendency to improve slowly over several months or a year or two. The only medications which have been shown to be of any benefit in chronic bronchopulmonary dysplasia are:

- Oxygen, if the infant is hypoxic
- Good nutrition, to improve muscle strength
- Diuretics, since some degree of fluid overload seems to contribute to the airway obstruction
- Traditionally, a combination of hydrochlorothiazide and spironolactone is used for these infants

Recurrent aspiration

Gastro-oesophageal reflux with aspiration of even small quantities of gastric contents is a potent cause of wheezing and the clinical picture may closely resemble bronchial asthma.

- Stopping all oral feeding and giving fluids intravenously for 2–3 days may help clarify the picture
- Medical anti-reflux treatment includes giving cisapride or omeprazole and alginic acid to thicken the feeds
- Infants or young children with reflux and aspiration causing signifant symptoms usually require surgical fundoplication

Cardiac failure

In some infants presenting with wheezing and COPD the source of the problem lies in the cardiovascular system; this complication is particularly common where there is a high pulmonary blood flow, which is often due to a relative simple anomaly such as with a patent ductus arteriosus or atrial septal defect.

- Bronchodilator or other medication for asthma is of no benefit but diuretics may help a little
- The infant will continue to wheeze until the cardiac problem is corrected

Congenital anomalies in children

Congenital anomalies of the airways and lungs or vascular rings compressing the airways are not responsive to medication. It is very common for such children to have received large amounts of medication for asthma and/or antibiotics for supposed pneumonia before the correct diagnosis is made. Management choice lies between surgery and simply following the child to see how he or she develops. If the child is feeding well, gaining weight well, not hypoxic and not severely distressed, it is usually best to avoid surgery.

Concerning vascular rings, most would take a conservative approach to incomplete rings if the child is thriving, but recommend surgery to open all types of complete ring, since these are very likely to become more problematic with growth.

Bronchodilators (relievers)

Relievers or bronchodilators give relatively rapid relief of symptoms and are believed to work predominantly by relaxation of airway smooth muscle (although several other effects on the airways may contribute to their anti-asthma effects). Relievers have no effect on the chronic inflammation of asthma.

Short-acting inhaled β_2-agonists

Mode of action

- β_2-receptors on airway smooth muscle: relaxation in large and small airways. Functional antagonists: reverse bronchoconstriction irrespective of cause
- Mast cell stabilizers (useful in protecting against allergen- and exercise-induced asthma)
- Experimentally reduce plasma exudation, reduce cholinergic reflexes
- Increase mucociliary clearance
- No effect on chronic inflammation in asthma

Recommended use

- Inhaled route always preferred. Oral route may be useful in infants with mild asthma
- Some believe they should not be used regularly (tolerance of protective effects, possible increase in morbidity and mortality)
- Prevention of exercise-induced asthma

Side-effects

- Muscle tremor (direct effect on skeletal muscle β_2-receptors). More common in elderly patients but does occur sometimes in children
- Tachycardia (direct effect on atrial β_2-receptors, reflex effect from increased peripheral vasodilatation via β_2-receptors)
- Hypokalaemia (direct effect on skeletal muscle uptake of K+ via β_2-receptors). Usually a small effect
- Restlessness – may be very troublesome in some infants
- Hypoxaemia (increased ventilation/perfusion mismatch due to pulmonary vasodilatation)
- Worsening of asthma control? (controversial: probably only applies to very high doses)

The choice and doses of short-acting β_2-agonists is described in the Appendix.

Long-acting inhaled β_2-agonists

These include salmeterol and formoterol. Both give bronchodilatation and protection against bronchoconstriction for >12 hours.

Clinical use

- As regular bronchodilators in children not well controlled taking low-dose inhaled steroids before increasing the dose of inhaled steroids
- Useful in nocturnal asthma (single night-time dose sometimes useful)
- Prolonged protection against exercise-induced asthma (most effective when not used on a regular basis)
- No anti-inflammatory effect alone, therefore *always* use in combination with an inhaled steroid when given continuously for prophylaxis

Theophylline

Classified as a bronchodilator, but relatively high doses needed for airway smooth muscle relaxation. There is now increasing evidence that theophylline has anti-inflammatory or immunomodulatory effects at lower plasma concentrations (5–10 mg/l). The drug can only be given orally.

Mode of action

- Phosphodiesterase inhibition (increases cyclic AMP and cyclic GMP levels)
- Adenosine receptor antagonism (accounts for some side-effects but little evidence that relevant for anti-asthma effects)
- Increased adrenaline secretion (but increase unlikely to account for anti-asthma effects)
- Prostaglandin inhibition
- Inhibition of calcium entry/release or phosphoinositide hydrolysis
- Unknown: difficult to explain all of the anti-asthma effects of theophylline on above mechanisms, as many only occur at concentrations higher than those used therapeutically

Recommended use

- As additional bronchodilator in children not well controlled taking low-dose inhaled steroids before increasing the dose of inhaled steroids
- Useful in nocturnal asthma as single night-time dose. Oral route of administration advantageous for some children
- Slow-release theophylline preparations have been popular as first-line prophylactic agents for asthma especially in USA
- Give either once or twice daily in dose to give plasma theophylline concentration of 5–10 mg/l

Side-effects

- Nausea and vomiting
- Headache
- Restlessness – very troublesome in infants and young children
- Gastroesophageal reflux
- Diuresis – may result in return of bed-wetting
- Cardiac arrythmias (usually plasma concentration >20 mg/l)
- Epileptic seizures (usually plasma concentration >30 mg/l)
- Learning disturbance in children (controversial)

Clearance of theophylline

The therapeutic effect is related to the plasma concentration which is affected by several factors that alter clearance. With the new recommendations on dosage this is less likely to be a problem. The plasma concentration may need to be checked from time to time.

Anticholinergics

The most commonly used anticholinergics are ipratropium bromide (MDI or nebulizer preparations available) and oxitropium bromide (MDI preparation only).

Mode of action

- Muscarinic receptor antagonists
- Inhibit cholinergic reflex bronchoconstriction
- Reduce vagal cholinergic tone

Recommended use

- In combination with β_2-agonist in treatment of acute asthma attack
- Additional bronchodilator in children taking high-dose inhaled steroids
- Some recommend use in infants as first-line bronchodilator
- Useful in COPD (e.g. BPD, CF) as vagal tone is the major reversible component)

Side-effects

- Bitter taste
- Systemic effects e.g. dry mouth, urinary retention, constipation (very rare)

Controllers

The term 'controller' is used for treatments that suppress the underlying inflammatory process in asthmatic airways. The previously used term 'anti-inflammatory treatment' is unsatisfactory as there are several types of inflammation. Thus, β_2-agonists are anti-inflammatory in the sense that they inhibit the release of inflammatory mediators from mast cells, yet they do not reduce the chronic inflammation in asthmatic airways (as measured in bronchial biopsies). Glucocorticoids are the only drugs that have been shown significantly to reduce the inflammation in asthmatic airways.

Inhaled steroids

Inhaled steroids are now introduced at a much earlier stage in treatment and are becoming the controllers of choice in the management of children with asthma.

Mode of action

- Bind to cytosolic glucocorticoid receptors that regulate the expression of multiple genes
- Inhibit the synthesis of multiple cytokines involved in asthmatic inflammation, such as IL-5, thus reducing eosinophilic infiltration into airways
- Inhibit the production of other inflammatory mediators, such as leukotrienes and prostaglandins
- Inhibit plasma exudation and mucus secretion
- Increase expression of airway β_2-receptors and prevent desensitization of β_2-receptors
- Prevent tissue remodelling?

Clinical efficacy

- Effective in virtually all children, irrespective of age or severity of asthma
- Reduce asthma symptoms (usually within days)
- Improve lung function (over days to weeks)
- Reduce airway hyper-responsiveness (though not usually back to normal). Improvement occurs slowly over several months
- Reduce frequency of asthma attacks and hospital admissions
- Reduce asthma mortality?
- May prevent irreversible airway narrowing in children
- Effects reverse when stopped (i.e. steroids suppress inflammation but do not cure its underlying cause)

Recommended use

- Use in any child taking a short-acting inhaled β_2-agonist more than once daily
- Use in any child with chronic perennial asthma not being controlled by prophylaxis with sodium cromoglycate or theophylline
- Start at relatively high dose to establish effective control of asthma rapidly, then reduce to minimal dose needed over 6 months
- Use twice daily on a regular basis (at low doses, once daily may suffice). When asthma is unstable t.d.s. administration is preferable
- Systemic effects possible with very high doses
- Budesonide and fluticasone propionate preferable to beclomethasone dipropionate as fewer systemic effects
- Use a spacer with a low-resistance valve or a dry powder inhaler and recommend mouth-washing when high doses needed

Side-effects – local

- Much less common in children than in adults
- Due to deposition of inhaled steroid in the oropharynx
- Markedly reduced by use of a spacer with an MDI, or mouth-washing with a dry powder inhaler
- Hoarseness (dysphonia)
- Oropharyngeal candidiasis
- Throat irritation and cough (most likely to be due to additives in MDI; rarely occur with dry powder inhalers)

Side-effects – systemic

- Systemic side-effects are due to absorption of inhaled steroids from the gastrointestinal tract and the respiratory tract (Fig.10)
- The gastrointestinal fraction is markedly reduced by a spacer or mouth-washing
- It is less evident with budesonide and fluticasone which are rapidly metabolized by first-pass metabolism in the liver

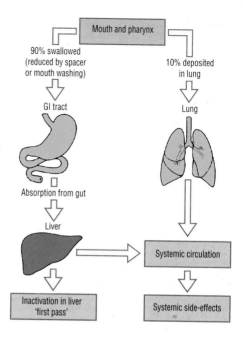

Figure 10

The fate of inhaled steroids. A large proportion of inhaled steroid is deposited in the mouth and pharynx and may be swallowed and absorbed from the gut. Systemic effects may arise from the fraction absorbed via the gut and liver into the systemic circulation, and from the fraction absorbed from the lung. Systemic effects can be markedly reduced by using a large volume spacer (for MDIs) to reduce oropharyngeal deposition or by mouth washing and discarding to prevent swallowing the deposited fraction (for DPIs).

There are many reports of systemic side-effects after inhaled steroids but these are often difficult to interpret as the patients had also received courses of systemic steroids. There are now several controlled trials measuring systemic effects of inhaled steroids using sensitive indices such as metabolic markers of bone metabolism (plasma osteocalcin, urinary pyridinium cross-links), short-term growth (knemometry) and suppression of adrenal function. Whether a small inhibitory effect in a very sensitive test is clinically relevant in terms of statural growth in children is not yet certain.

The following systemic side-effects of corticosteroids are recognized:

- Adrenal suppression
- Increased bone turnover, osteoporosis? (No evidence with inhaled corticosteroids)
- Cataracts? (no evidence with inhaled corticosteroids)
- Stunted growth in children? (not proven with inhaled corticosteroids in reasonable doses)
- Easy bruising (rare in children)
- Skin thinning (rare in children)
- Behavioural disturbances, such as hyperactivity
- Most studies have shown no clinically relevant systemic effects at daily doses of 400 µg of beclomethasone or budesonide in children

Growth and corticosteroids in childhood asthma

- Asthma itself may suppress growth by delaying bone maturation, so that growth may even accelerate when asthma is controlled
- A meta-analysis of 22 studies of growth in children treated with inhaled steroids has demonstrated no overall effect on growth or statural height
- Asthmatic children have about 15 months' delay on average in the onset of puberty which is unrelated to medication
- Steroid-taking adolescents may appear growth-retarded but will achieve their predicted height after puberty
- Systemic effects occur only in doses of >1600 µg daily of beclomethasone, budesonide or fluticasone and are fewer than observed with oral steroids, which are usually the only alternative therapy in severe disease

Cromones

Cromones include sodium cromoglycate (q.d.s. via MDI, nebulizer or DPI–Spinhaler and nedocromil sodium (t.d.s/q.d.s via MDI).

Mode of action

- Mast cell stabilization (however, other drugs with mast cell stabilizing properties are not effective in asthma)
- Inhibition of sensory nerve activation (effective in reducing cough)
- Inhibitory effect on several types of inflammatory cell (eosinophil, macrophages, neutrophils) in vitro
- Inhibit indirect bronchial challenges (allergen, exercise, cold air, SO_2, bradykinin) but no effect on direct challenges (histamine, methacholine)
- No convincing evidence for an anti-inflammatory effect in biopsy studies

Clinical efficacy

- Reduce asthma symptoms in some children with mild to moderate asthma. No obvious clinical indicators of patients who respond
- Some paediatricians prefer these drugs as first-line prophylaxis in children and only move on to inhaled steroids if they are not controlled
- Effective in preventing allergen- and exercise-induced symptoms if taken immediately prior to trigger (but not as effective as an inhaled β_2-agonist).
- May be given as nebulized form in infants
- Should be taken four times daily as short duration of action
- Less effective than inhaled steroids
- No evidence for additive effect with steroids and little evidence for useful steroid-sparing effect

Side-effects

- Extremely rare with cromoglycate
- Angioneurotic oedema (extremely rare)
- Coughing immediately after administration with dry powder (prevented by a β_2-agonist)
- Bitter taste (nedocromil only). Now available in menthol aerosols to mask taste
- Burning sensation (nedocromil only) due to activation of thermoreceptors

Oral steroids

Regular oral steroids are only indicated in the most severe asthmatic patients who cannot be controlled with high-dose inhaled steroids and additional regular bronchodilators, whereas short courses of oral steroids are commonly used to treat asthma exacerbations. Infants and young children quite unwilling to accept any form of inhaled steroids may need to be treated with oral steroids on a single-dose alternate morning basis.

The oral steroid of choice is *prednisolone* given as a single daily dose (usually in the morning) as this steroid has least systemic effects. Prednisolone is preferred to prednisone which has to be converted to prednisolone in the liver. In children on maintenance steroid therapy it is preferable to give alternate morning dosing, if possible, to reduce systemic side-effects.

Triamcinolone acetonide injections are a slow-release preparation of systemic steroids. Some patients who have poor compliance may be helped by this treatment given once monthly. There is a risk of developing proximal myopathy and systemic side-effects with this fluorinated steroid.

Short courses of oral steroids

- Indicated for exacerbations of asthma
- Course should normally last 5–7 days
- Reduce dose progressively after starting with about 2 mg/kg daily of prednisolone as a single morning dose

Maintenance oral steroids

- Use minimum dose needed to control asthma
- Use alternate-morning dosing if possible
- Reduce doses slowly if there is a risk of adrenal suppression
- Issue patient with a steroid card (and Medic-alert bracelet should be worn if possible)
- Increase dose if severe infection, major trauma, surgery, dental treatment

Side-effects

The side-effects of prolonged oral steroid therapy (more than 1–2 months) or frequent short course (more than once every 1–2 months for several months) are the same as for high doses of inhaled steroids with *in addition* the possibility of:

- Cushingoid appearance
- Increased weight (fluid retention and increased appetite)
- Osteoporosis, spontaneous fractures
- Stunted growth
- Gastrointestinal symptoms: dyspepsia, increase peptic ulceration
- Diabetes
- Hypertension
- Cataracts (postcapsular)
- Mental disturbance (euphoria, depression, mania)

Steroid-sparing therapies

In some patients, but rarely children who require maintenance oral steroids, serious side-effects such as growth stunting are an indication for introduction of a steroid-sparing therapy. These treatments usually have a high frequency of side-effects themselves and are therefore only indicated if the side-effects of oral steroids are a problem. These therapies have been shown in controlled trials of asthma to reduce prednisolone requirements by 5–10 mg daily, but are more effective in some patients than others.

Methotrexate

- Use low dose (7.5–17.5 mg total weekly, orally or i.m. have been used in children)
- Side-effects include nausea and vomiting (common, less if initial dose reduced), hepatic fibrosis, blood dyscrasias, opportunistic infections

Gold

- Small steroid-sparing effect
- Side-effects include renal damage (nephrotic syndrome), hepatic dysfunction

Cyclosporin A

- Active against CD4+ (helper) T-cells
- Has steroid-sparing effect in some patients in low dose (2–5 mg/kg daily has been used in adults)
- Side-effects include renal damage, hepatic dysfunction
- Monitor creatinine, liver function and blood pressure (check blood level)

Other therapies

> **Ketotifen**
> - Antihistamine with sedative effects
> - Controlled trials show little, if any, beneficial effect in children
>
> **Antihistamines**
> - Not clinically useful in controlling asthma symptoms
> - Nonsedative antihistamines (terfenadine, astemizole, loratadine) useful for concomitant rhinitis
>
> **Nonsteroidal anti-inflammatory drugs**
> - No beneficial effect and may cause exacerbation of symptoms in patients with aspirin-sensitive asthma
>
> **Immunotherapy**
> - Of little proven value
> - Side-effects (local reactions and anaphylaxis) outweigh any benefit
> - More effective therapies (medication) available
>
> **Calcium antagonists**
> - No beneficial effect in clinical asthma
>
> **Alpha-adrenergic antagonists**
> - No proven value in treatment of asthma symptoms
>
> **Anti leukotrienes**
> - LTD4 antagonists (zafirlukast and montelukast) and 5-lipoxygenase inhibitors (zileuton) are already being used in clinical practice. Paediatric clinical trials are awaited with great interest

Other treatments used in COPD of childhood

In addition to relievers and controllers, other treatments are used in non-asthma COPD and wheezing diseases.

Mucolytics

There is little evidence that mucolytics (acetylcysteine, carbocisteine, bromhexine) are useful in the treatment of diseases such as CF and bronchiolitis where there is increased production of sputum.

DNAse

Human recombinant DNAse (dornase-alpha, Pulmozyme) may benefit some patients with CF. DNA in sputum derived from bacteria and cellular debris results in a marked increase in sputum viscosity in CF. DNAse, when given by jet nebulization once daily, breaks down this DNA and reduces sputum viscosity, improving the ability to clear the airways. This results in a small increase in lung function and a reduced number of infective exacerbations. Not all patients benefit: the improvement is often small, and treatment is expensive. A trial of therapy over 4 weeks is therefore recommended and only patients showing significant clinical improvement should be maintained on this therapy. Side-effects are uncommon, but include pharyngitis and skin rashes.

Antibiotics

Broad-spectrum antibiotics are indicated for the treatment of infective exacerbations in CF and other diseases where bacterial infection is common, including structural problems with retention of secretions. These antibiotics need to be active against the likely organism and, in CF, *Pseudomonas spp* is common which is resistant to many antibiotics. Nebulized colomycin and oral ciprofloxacin are useful for treating exacerbations and for prevention. Intravenous antibiotics are often required for severe infective exacerbations (azlocillin, gentomicin, tobramycin or ceftazadime). Prophylactic antibiotics may be indicated in some patients with frequent exacerbations but the development of resistance may be a problem. Antibiotics are of no value in asthma other than to treat secondary infection such as may occur with obstruction of the middle lobe bronchus ('middle lobe syndrome').

Oxygen

Oxygen is indicated for the treatment of acute exacerbations of wheezing disorders when there is evidence of hypoxia. Chronic administration of oxygen at home may be indicated in patients with severe chronic airflow obstruction and is commonly used in hypoxic infants during the prolonged recovery from bronchopulmonary dysplasia.

Drug delivery systems

Wheezing diseases of infancy and childhood involve airway narrowing as a result of a combination of bronchospasm, inflammatory infiltration and secretion into the lumen. The most obvious and direct route for delivering drugs to the asthmatic airway is by inhalation and this route increases the local deposition while minimizing systemic effects. Fortunately, most of the medications needed to treat asthma can be delivered by inhalation. Other routes of medication, particularly oral and intravenous therapy may be more appropriate under some circumstances.

Inhaled route recommended for:

- β_2-agonists (except in some infants)
- Anticholinergics (always)
- Cromones (always)
- Corticosteroid prophylaxis (except in the severest unresponsive asthma)
- DNAse in cystic fibrosis
- Antibiotics in treatment of infective exacerbations in cystic fibrosis

Oral route recommended for:

- β_2-agonists in some infants with mild asthma
- Theophylline preparations for prophylaxis (always)
- Corticosteroids for relief of acute attacks (short 'crash' course)
- Corticosteroid prophylaxis in small children or others unable to use inhalers
- Corticosteroid prophylaxis of severe asthma unresponsive to inhaled steroids

Intravenous route recommended for:

- Corticosteroids for treatment of status asthmaticus (if unwilling or unable to take oral steroids)
- Aminophylline if indicated for status asthmaticus
- β_2-agonists if indicated for status asthmaticus (rarely necessary)

Intramuscular route recommended for:

- Depot corticosteroids for asthma uncontrolled by other methods (rarely indicated)

Administration of medications by inhalation

Given the central role of inhalation therapy for most asthma treatment it is important to understand the way in which different delivery systems work and how they should be used by the patient. *Unless the physician understands the use of an inhaler device and can use it effectively it is highly unlikely that his or her patients will do so*. There are four basic systems currently available for delivering drugs by inhalation (Fig. 11).

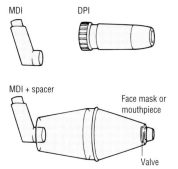

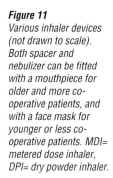

Figure 11
Various inhaler devices (not drawn to scale). Both spacer and nebulizer can be fitted with a mouthpiece for older and more co-operative patients, and with a face mask for younger or less co-operative patients. MDI= metered dose inhaler, DPI= dry powder inhaler.

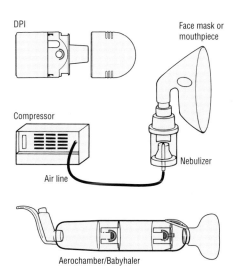

Metered dose inhaler (MDI)

The MDI contains medication mixed with a chlorofluorocarbon (CFC) propellant (soon to be replaced by a hydrofluorocarbon which has less effect on the ozone layer) and a controlled dose is emitted as a spray when the device is activated. It is a very convenient delivery system and MDIs are available for all commonly available asthma medications except theophylline preparations.

Metered dose inhaler (MDI)

Advantages
- Small and portable
- Cheap
- Quick to use

Disadvantages
- Perfect technique essential
- Unsuitable for children <5–6 years
- Cold jet may irritate throat
- CFCs may damage ozone layer

Correct technique
- Shake the inhaler
- Hold upright
- Breathe out
- Close lips around mouthpiece
- Fire device at start of slow inspiration
- Inspire to total lung capacity
- Hold breath for 10 seconds
- Breathe out

When the treatment calls for two or more doses of medication it is important that each dose be taken separately and it is not recommended to actuate the MDI more than once per inspiration.

Metered dose inhaler (MDI) with spacer

Because many patients, both young and old, are unable to coordinate well enough to use an MDI correctly, various holding chambers (spacers) have been developed which are placed between the MDI and the patient. The drug is inhaled from the chamber and coordination with the firing of the MDI is no longer important. Most spacers have some type of one-way valve. Some are large volume, some much smaller, and there are spacers with face masks suitable for infants. The type of spacer used is probably of little importance in most cases, providing the physician makes certain that the infant or child will obtain the inhaled medication reliably.

Metered dose inhaler (MDI) with spacer

Advantages
- Coordination unimportant
- Can be used for all ages
- May reduce systemic absorption (important for corticosteroids)
- May be effective even in severe asthma (high doses can be given)
- Relatively inexpensive

Disadvantages
- Bulky and inconvenient
- Valves sometimes stick or become incompetent
- CFCs may damage ozone layer

Correct technique
- Shake the inhaler
- Fix MDI upright in spacer
- Keep lips on mouthpiece or keep face mask tightly applied to face (infants)
- Breathe in and out through spacer
- Fire device while taking 3–4 deep breaths
- Be sure valve is operating
- Keep spacer clean and dry (but do not wash too often as inhaled drug more likely to stick to chamber walls)

When the treatment calls for two or more doses of medication it is important that each dose be taken separately and it is not recommended to load the spacer with several doses.

Dry powder inhaler (DPI)

While one type of powder inhaler (Spinhaler) has been available for many years, a number of newer multidose devices have been developed from which the patient inhales a dry powder formulation of the drug. These do not contain CFCs and since they are only activated by the inspiratory effort of the patient coordination is not a problem, although the inhalation technique is still very important. Multidose types of powder inhalers are suitable for most patients including those who would require a spacer in order to use an MDI.

Dry powder inhaler (DPI)	
Advantages	**Disadvantages**
• Coordination unimportant	• More expensive than MDI
• Can be used for most children over 5 years	• Requires rapid inspiration
• Small and portable	
• No CFCs	
• Multidose dry powder devices (Turbuhaler, Diskhaler, Accuhaler) convenient, easy to operate	

Correct technique
• Follow instructions for preparation of device
• Breathe out
• Place lips firmly around mouthpiece
• Breathe in rapidly and deeply

Nebulizer

Jet nebulizers produce a cloud of medication by passing a jet of compressed air over a solution of the drug. They require a compressor (electric or battery-operated) or a source of gas (air or oxygen). *Ultrasonic nebulizers* produce the cloud by vibration of a plate at high frequency onto which the solution is dropped.

Preparations of bronchodilators (β_2-agonists, anticholinergics), sodium cromoglycate and steroids (budesonide only) are available for nebulization. Nebulizers are also used for administering antibiotics, DNAse and other mucolytics.

Nebulizer	
Advantages	**Disadvantages**
• Coordination unimportant	• Cumbersome equipment
• Can be used for all ages	• Expensive and noisy
• Effective in severe asthma	• Treatment takes a long time
• No CFCs	• Disliked by some infants, loathed by others
• Needed for delivery of antibiotics, DNAse	• May deliver too high doses of drug

Correct technique
- Follow instructions for preparation of device
- Breathe normally through mouthpiece or face mask
- Breathe continuously for at least 5–6 minutes

Dose of inhaled medications

The actual dose of medication reaching the lungs from most inhalation devices is only about 10% of that nominally delivered by the device, whether it be an MDI, DPI or nebulizer, and in many situations it is even less. Much of the drug is impacted on the device itself and some particles are too large to reach the lungs and impact on the buccal mucosa with the potential for systemic absorption. This is particularly important for inhaled steroids and there are some data to suggest that the use of a spacer reduces this unwanted effect. Even though the lung dose is relatively low, drug delivery by inhalation is usually highly effective if the correct inhalation technique is used. The Turbuhaler appears to deliver about twice as much medication as the equivalent MDI and the dose may need to be reduced accordingly.

Which inhalation device for which patient?

Infants and children up to 5 years	MDI + spacer, Nebulizer
Children 5–9 years	MDI (?), MDI + spacer, DPI, Nebulizer
Competent older children	MDI, DPI
Incompetent older children	MDI + spacer, Nebulizer (?)

Education of child, family and other carers

The successful management of asthma largely depends on providing the child and those with responsibility for its care with a good understanding of the nature of asthma and its treatment. The physician must take time to explain this to the child and the parents in terms that they can understand, and the message must be reinforced at subsequent visits. There are a number of important points that should be made:

- There is no cure for asthma but there is excellent treatment which can allow virtually all asthmatics to lead normal lives. Almost all children become completely symptom-free or almost symptom-free during or by the end of childhood. There is some evidence that good treatment encourages this tendency to grow out of asthma
- Asthma is rarely fatal but, in those cases where it is, there has almost always been inadequate treatment or failure to comply with medical advice. Children do not need to be over-protected because they have asthma but parents need to appreciate problems when they arise
- Far more patients die because they do not get corticosteroid therapy than the reverse. In conventional doses, corticosteroids are not harmful to children and they form the mainstay of the treatment of serious chronic asthma at all ages
- Compliance with treatment is essential. The major causes of inadequate control of asthma and consequent suffering are the three big Fs:

Cont'd.

FAILURE TO TAKE PRESCRIBED MEDICATIONS REGULARLY

FAILURE TO TAKE THE PRESCRIBED DOSE

FAILURE TO USE INHALERS PROPERLY

The physician should make every attempt to verify compliance with treatment at each visit and should always check on inhaler technique and the functioning of spacer devices. The child should be taught to assume responsibility for their own treatment as much as possible, commensurate with age and understanding.

The simpler the regimen, the more likely is patient and family compliance and successful control of asthma.

Ancillary devices to aid management

Given the fact that the management of asthma is ambulatory for most patients almost all of the time, the physician often needs objective information on the condition of the child while engaged in normal activities. The parents also need to know what to do about treatment without consulting the physician at every turn. A number of ancillary devices have been developed for these purposes.

Diary cards (Fig. 12)

Diary cards are the simplest and possibly the most useful device, providing a daily record of symptoms and drug consumption. They are particularly useful when evaluating a new patient, or when changing treatment regimens.

Action plans (Fig. 13)

An extension of the diary is to provide the patient with a written 'action plan'. This should be as simple as possible, occupying no more than one typed sheet. It should only involve PEF measurements if it is certain that this is necessary and will be undertaken properly by the child.

Year *1997* Month *August*	Day	1	2	3	4	5	6
Nighttime or early morning cough / wheeze	None 0 Mild 1 Moderate 2 Severe 3	0	1	2	2	1	0
Daytime cough / wheeze	None 0 Mild 1 Moderate 2 Severe 3	0	0	0	2	2	0
Limitation of activity or exercise	None 0 Mild 1 Moderate 2 Severe 3	0	0	0	2	2	0
Controller medications Name (strength) *Pulmicort (200)*	Doses / day taken	2	1	2	2	2	2
Reliever medications Name (strength) *Ventolin (100)*	Doses / day taken	0	0	3	4	3	1
Morning PEF Evening PEF	Best of three Best of three						
Comments							

Figure 12
Diary for recording asthma symptoms, peak flow and medications, suitable for both children and adults.

The action plan should contain the following elements:

- Name and telephone number of all treating physicians/hospitals
- Usual regular medications with exact doses and instructions for their use
- Simple extra medications (bronchodilators) to be used when needed
- Emergency medications/action to be taken when needed
- Expected condition when well-controlled, based on symptoms
- Indications for simple extra medication, based on symptoms
- Indication for emergency treatment, based on symptoms
- How to step down treatment when condition improves

ASTHMA ACTION PLAN	SYMPTOMS	TREATMENT

ASTHMA ACTION PLAN

Name _____
GP _____ Tel _____
Hospital doctor _____
                  Tel _____

Reliever medication:
name _____
strength _____
doses per day _____

Controller medication:
name _____
strength _____
doses per day _____

Emergency prednisolone
starting dose _____
duration _____

SYMPTOMS	TREATMENT
Feel fine	No change in treatment
Waking at night cough / wheeze by day	Take more reliever
Getting worse despite reliever	Double dose of preventer
No better or breathless at rest	Start course of prednisolone
Getting worse or needing reliever every 1–2 hours	Call ambulance Continue reliever

Figure 13
Simple action plan suitable for paediatric patients without reference to peak flow recording.

Who should take care of the patient, and where?

Asthma is a common disease in children and most sufferers are only mildly affected. For these patients, excellent care can be provided by the general practitioner or primary care paediatrician. The difficult questions arise when control is not good and the child is limited in normal everyday activities, or when they appear to be resistant to acceptable doses of usual medication. In such patients it is worth obtaining the opinion of an expert in paediatric respiratory medicine. Once the child has been stabilized, further supervision will depend upon the circumstances and experience of the various physicians involved. The potential for serious side-effects means that most steroid-dependent children should be seen at a specialist clinic.

The patient should be sent straight to the Accident and Emergency Department if:

- The patient has bad asthma which is getting worse, despite treatment
- The patient is cyanosed or drowsy
- The patient is scared
- The doctor is scared!

Schooling and the asthmatic child

With proper management, asthma should cause little or no interference with schooling in the large majority of children. They should be able to take part in all normal activities, including games and competitive sports. However, some children on three-times-daily prophylactic medication (usually sodium cromoglycate) will need to take their medication at school, and others may need to take their as-needed β_2-agonist from time to time and especially before physical exercise.

How teachers (or other carers) should deal with the asthmatic pupil

Teachers should:

- Know which children in their class have asthma
- Understand the nature of asthma and its treatment
- Know that exercise can be difficult for the asthmatic
- Know that asthmatics may need to take a β_2-agonist before exercise
- Know how asthma medications are taken, especially inhaled β_2-agonists
- Recognize deteriorating asthma and inform the parents
- Know how to give inhaled medications for an acute attack
- Strongly discourage cigarette smoking by children, parents and teachers

---

Additional therapeutic approaches

Several non-pharmacological approaches have been used in the treatment of wheezing disorders in children. These often have little or no efficacy, but may have a useful placebo effect. It is important that introduction of alternative therapies is not accompanied by withdrawal of conventional therapies.

Allergen avoidance

Since most childhood asthma is allergic in nature, allergen avoidance is a logical approach. It is difficult to avoid completely exposure to allergens, even using the most rigorous avoidance measures. Nevertheless, several controlled trials have demonstrated some improvement in asthma control and simple avoidance measures are worth trying:

House dust mite avoidance
- Mattress and pillow barrier covers (expensive)
- Use terylene/foam filling for pillows and duvets; avoid feathers
- No carpet or curtains in the bedroom (linoleum floor, blinds preferable)
- Frequent vacuum cleaning and damp dusting of bedrooms
- Put soft toys in deep freeze every week
- Acaricide sprays not effective

Grass pollen avoidance
- Avoid walking in parks or fields during pollen season
- Keep bedroom windows closed during pollen season

Cat/furry pet avoidance
- Remove cats from the home if possible (but allergen may persist for months)
- Washing cat probably *not* effective
- Never allow cat to sleep on the bed

Diet

Many parents believe that dietary factors, especially milk, worsen asthma. Except in rare instances of true cow's milk protein allergic asthma, there is no evidence to support this belief. Food additives, such as sodium metabisulphite and tartrazine, may worsen asthma and should be avoided when this is the case. There is little evidence that asthma is triggered by an allergic reaction to foods, but a trial of avoidance of the suspected food may sometimes be worthwhile.

There is some evidence that a reduced intake of antioxidants (vitamins C and E, beta-carotene) and fish, and an increased intake of salt, are associated with increased asthma prevalence. A healthy, balanced diet is therefore recommended. Dietary supplements may be indicated in cystic fibrosis where there is significant malnutrition due to malabsorption. Many infants with severe COPD are malnourished, and the improvement of nutritional status seems to be important in aiding recovery. This may even require a feeding gastrostomy if oral supplementation is impractical.

Hypnosis and complementary medicine

There is no convincing evidence from controlled trials that hypnosis or complementary medical techniques are helpful in the management of asthma.

Appendix: Dosages

The dosages recommended in this book are in accordance with those recommended in the British National Formulary, modified in the light of the author's experience where necessary. Care is always needed when prescribing for children and the reader must personally verify the doses of medications prescribed.

Regular maintenance medication

Bronchodilators	
Salbutamol	*Syrup* for small children: 0.15 mg/kg/dose (max 3 mg) up to four times daily
	Nebulizer solution (5 mg/ml): 0.5 ml diluted to 2–3 ml up to four times daily
	MDI (100 µg/puff) with or without spacer: 1–2 puffs as needed up to four times daily
	Dry powder inhaler (Diskhaler) – (200 or 400 µg): 1–2 as needed up to four times daily

Terbutaline	*Syrup* for small children: 0.15 mg/kg/dose (max 3 mg) up to four times daily
	Nebulizer solution (10 mg/ml): 0.5 ml diluted to 2–3 ml up to four times daily
	MDI (250 µg/puff) with or without spacer: 1–2 puffs as needed up to four times daily
	Dry powder inhaler (Turbuhaler) (500 µg/dose): one inhalation up to four times daily
Salmeterol	Long-acting β_2-agonist for regular use
	MDI (25 µg/puff): 1–2 puffs twice daily
	Dry powder inhaler (Diskhaler) (50 µg/puff): 1–2 puffs twice daily
Eformoterol	Long-acting β_2-agonist for regular use
	Dry powder inhaler (12 g/capsule): 1–2 capsules twice daily
Other β_2-agonists	These are used less often:
	Fenoterol, pirbuterol, reproterol, orciprenaline, rimiterol
	Note: It is not recommended to prescribe regular daily short-acting β_2-agonist medication on a long-term basis and these drugs should be used primarily as rescue medication. Salmeterol should only be used in combination with inhaled steroids
Ipratropium bromide	Anticholinergic bronchodilator, less effective than β-agonists in routine asthma treatment
	Nebulizer solution (0.25 mg/ml): 0.25–1.00 ml three to four times daily
	MDI (20/40 µg/puff): 1–2 puffs three to four times daily
Oxitropium bromide	*MDI* (100 µg/puff): 2 puffs three times daily

Controllers	
Sodium cromoglycate	*Nebulizer solution*: 20 mg (2 ml) three to four times daily as prophylaxis
	Powder inhaler (Spinhaler): 20 mg three to four times daily as prophylaxis
	MDI (1 or 5 mg/puff): 1–2 puffs four times daily as prophylaxis
Nedocromil sodium	*MDI (2 mg/puff)*: 2 puffs two to four times daily as prophylaxis
Slow-release theophylline preparations	Many preparations as prophylaxis • *Children*: build up to about 5 mg/kg twice daily with checks on blood level • *Adults*: build up to about 4 mg/kg twice daily with checks on blood level These doses are designed to give blood levels in the range of 5–10 mg/litre

Inhaled steroids	
Low-dose: total daily dose	Beclomethasone dipropionate (BDP) or budesonide: <400 μg in children (800 μg in adults) Fluticasone propionate (FP): <200 μg in children (400 μg in adults)
High dose: total daily dose	BDP or budesonide: 400–1000 μg in children (800–2000 μg in adults) FP: 200–500 μg in children (400–1000 μg in adults) • Dose delivered to lungs depends on delivery device • Daily dose determined by asthma severity; use lowest dose needed to maintain control • Twice daily administration recommended
Beclomethasone dipropionate	*MDI* (50, 100, 200 and 250 μg/puff) *Dry powder inhaler* (100, 200, 400 μg/dose)

Budesonide	MDI (50 and 200 µg/puff)
	Dry powder inhaler (Turbuhaler) (100 and 400 µg/inhalation). Data suggest that dose should be about half that for the MDI preparation but individual adjustment will be necessary
	Nebulized (250 and 500 µg/ml; 0.5–1.0 mg b.d.)
Fluticasone propionate	MDI (25, 50, 125 and 250 µg/puff)
	Dry powder inhaler (50, 100, 250 µg/dose)
	Twice as potent as beclomethasone and budesonide

Oral steroids	
Use lowest dose possible for maintenance therapy	Children: use alternate-morning single dose (average maintenance dose up to 1 mg/kg of prednisolone/alternate mornings)
	Adults: give as single morning dose
Prednisolone	(1 and 5 mg; enteric-coated tablets also available)
Betamethasone	(0.5 mg tablets) approximately 10 times as potent as prednisolone

Short (crash) course of corticosteroids

Children: Oral prednisolone – start with 2.0 mg/kg/day in divided doses and reduce in steps to zero over 5–10 days provided control is adequate. If not, consider higher dose or longer course but courses lasting more than 2–3 weeks are likely to cause side-effects.

Acute (emergency) medications

Bronchodilators	
Salbutamol	*Nebulized:* *Children*: 0.15 mg/kg up to 5.0 mg maximum diluted to 2–3 ml with normal saline *Adults:* 5.0 mg diluted to 2–3 ml with normal saline *MDI*: *Both:* 20 puffs of MDI into large-volume spacer *Intravenous*: *Children*: 0.1–0.2 µg/kg/min *Adults*: initially 5 µg/min, then adjust to avoid excessive heart rate response (average dose 3–20 µg/min)
Terbutaline	*Nebulized:* *Children*: 0.3 mg/kg up to 10.0 mg maximum diluted to 2–3 ml with normal saline *Adults*: 10 mg diluted to 2–3 ml with normal saline *MDI*: *Both:* 20 puffs of MDI into large-volume spacer *Intravenous:* *Children*: 0.02–0.06 µg/kg/min *Adults*: 1.5–5.0 µg/min
Ipratropium bromide	*Nebulized*: To be added to β$_2$-agonist inhalation every 2–4 hours *Children*: 5–7 µg/kg *Adults*: 500 mg (2.0 ml of 250 µg/ml solution)
Aminophylline	If patient has *not* been taking theophylline preparations: loading dose of 7 mg/kg up to maximum of 250 mg over 20 minutes then maintenance of 0.5–1.0 mg/kg/h and measure blood level If patient *has* been taking theophylline preparations: no loading dose, only maintenance of 0.5–1.0 mg/kg/h and measure blood level

Corticosteroids

Oral prednisolone	*Children*: give 2 mg/kg stat, then tail down over 7–10 days *Adults*: give 60 mg stat then tail down over 7–10 days
Intravenous hydrocortisone	*Children*: 4.0 mg/kg every 6 h *Adults*: 200 mg every 6 h
Intravenous methylpred-nisolone	*Children*: 1.0–1.5 mg/kg every 6 h *Adults*: 100 mg every 6 h

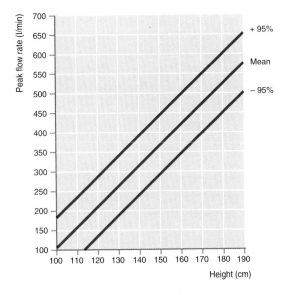

Figure 14
This nomogram results from tests carried out by Professor S Godfrey and his colleagues on a sample of 382 normal boys and girls aged 5–18 years. Each child blew five times into a standard Wright Peak Flow Meter and the highest reading was accepted in each case. All measurements were completed within a six-week period. The outer lines of the graph indicated that the results of 95% of the children fell within these boundaries. (Redrawn from Godfrey et al. Br J Dis Chest *(1970)* **64**: 15.)

Further reading

Asthma: a follow-up statement from an international paediatric asthma consensus group. *Arch Dis Child* 1992; **67**: 240–8.

Barnes PJ, Leff AR, Grunstein M, Woolcock A. *Asthma*. Philadelphia: Lippincott-Raven, 1996.

British Thoracic Society et al. Guidelines on the management of asthma. *Thorax* 1993; **48** (suppl): S1–S48.

Global Strategy for Asthma Management and Prevention. NHLBI/WHO Workshop Report (95-3659) 1995.

Godfrey S. Selected topics in respiratory medicine: Bronchiolitis and asthma in infancy and early childhood. *Thorax* 1996; **51** (suppl 2): S60–S64.

Chernick V, Kendig EL Jr. *Kendig's Disorders of the Respiratory Tract in Children*. Philadelphia: WB Saunders Company, 1990.

National Heart, Lung and Blood Institute, National Institutes of Health. International consensus report on the diagnosis and management of asthma. *Eur Respir J* 1992; **5**: 601–41.

Phelan PD, Landau LI, Olonsky A. *Respiratory Illnesses in Children*. Oxford: Blackwell Scientific Publications, 1982.

Index

Page numbers in *italic* refer to the illustrations